COOKIE DIET

Maintaining a Healthy Diet: A Comprehensive Overview of Cookie Diet Meals

CARL JUAN

Table of Contents

Introductory

One method of dieting known as the "Cookie Diet" entails subsisting primarily (or entirely) on cookies of a specific kind. with order to aid with hunger control and calorie reduction, these cookies are often made with a high fiber and protein content and a low calorie count.

• The idea behind the Cookie Diet is that by replacing regular meals with these cookies, dieters can cut back on calories without feeling deprived. The idea is that the cookies give a handy and portion-controlled solution to regulate calorie intake.

• One of the more well-known Cookie Diet plans was created by Dr. Sanford Siegal, a Miami-based physician. His cookies have been sold as "Dr. Siegal's Cookie Diet" in an effort to assist people reduce their body mass. Warning: the Cookie Diet is too restricted to be a long-term solution to your weight problem. Cookies are delicious, but they probably won't provide the balanced diet necessary for long-term health if that's all you eat.

• While the Cookie Diet's low-calorie eating plan may help some people lose weight in the short term, it's not a sustainable solution.

Adopting a varied diet, engaging in regular physical activity, and working with a healthcare practitioner to set realistic goals is a more sustainable and balanced approach to weight management.

CHAPTER ONE
The Science behind the Cookie Diet

The Cookie Diet, commonly known as "Dr. Siegel's Cookie Diet," is a weight control plan based on replacing regular cookies with specially prepared ones. This is how the diet usually goes down:

• The Cookie Diet calls for the substitution of specially formulated, low-calorie cookies for regular meals like breakfast, lunch, and snacks. These cookies are intended to be used as a meal replacement.

• **Calorie Reduction:** Each cookie has between 90 and 120 calories, depending on the specific recipe. Eating fewer calories, such as those included in these cookies, is a fundamental component of slimming down.

• Calorie consumption at each meal is set in advance thanks to the cookies' portion control feature. This can be useful for controlling hunger and limiting calorie consumption.

• Cookies are often made with a high protein and fiber content to help curb hunger and make you feel fuller for longer. This, in turn, can help you eat less and snack less frequently.

- Supplement with a Balanced Dinner: Many variants of the Cookie Diet permit participants to consume a healthy, well-balanced dinner each night. Lean protein, vegetables, and a few carbs make up the bulk of this meal. The goal is to create a more well-rounded diet.

- Drinking enough of water is recommended on the Cookie Diet since it can aid with satiety and general health.

- Check-ins with a health care provider or a weight loss coach are a component of some variations of the Cookie Diet in order to keep track of progress and offer emotional support.

It's crucial to note that while the Cookie Diet may contribute to immediate weight loss owing to reduced calorie consumption, it is considered a highly restricted and potentially unsustainable strategy to weight control. The risks and restrictions of this diet include the following:

Relying solely on cookies as a source of nutrition might lead to nutritional inadequacies.

The Cookie Diet is typically seen as a quick fix, however it may not instill healthy eating patterns that can last.

There isn't much to eat, so the diet could get boring quickly.

There is a risk of relying too heavily on processed meals.

If you want to lose weight safely and effectively, it's best to talk to a doctor or a trained dietitian before beginning any program, including the Cookie Diet. You can learn to manage your weight in a more healthy and long-lasting way with their assistance.

The Weight Loss Benefits of Cookies

It's not common to associate cookies, especially the kind you get from the bakery that's loaded with sugar, white flour, and butter. In reality, these cookies tend to be high in sugar, bad fats, and calories, making them a terrible choice for dieters. There are, however, some cookie varieties and diet plans that are designed to aid in weight loss. Here's how cookies aid in shedding pounds:

1. Meal Replacement Cookies: Some weight loss programs offer specially created meal replacement cookies that are supposed to be low in calories, sugar, and bad fats. By substituting these cookies for regular meals, you can cut back on calories and maybe even lose some weight because of their portion control, convenience, and low calorie count. Meal replacement cookies are a convenient and healthy alternative to traditional meals.

2. Cookies, when eaten in moderation and as part of a healthy diet, can aid in controlling food intake. Small, portion-controlled cookies are a great way to satisfy a

sweet taste without going overboard on calories.

3. Some people use their ingenuity and ingredients like whole-grain flour, oats, and natural sweeteners like honey or maple syrup to create healthier cookie alternatives. If you're trying to watch your sugar and fat intake, these baked goods can be made with less sugar and better fats.

4. Traditional cookies aren't the best choice if you're trying to trim down, but they may still be a part of a healthy diet if you keep the portions in check. For successful long-term weight management, it may be helpful to indulge in little portions of your favorite foods on a regular basis.

• Whether you're included them in your diet or enjoying them as a treat, cookies belong in the context of a healthy, varied, and balanced meal plan. Even "healthy" or "weight loss" cookies, if eaten in excess, can lead to weight gain for the same reasons as eating regular cookies.

For effective and permanent weight loss, it's recommended to focus on a diet that includes a range of nutritious foods, such as fruits, vegetables, lean proteins, whole grains, and healthy fats, while also including regular physical activity. If you want to lose weight in a healthy and safe way, consulting with a licensed dietician or healthcare expert can help.

CHAPTER TWO
The Cookie Diet: Getting Ready

There are a number of things you can do to increase your chances of success on the Cookie Diet or another meal replacement plan that involves eating specially made cookies. To help you get ready, here are some suggestions:

1. Meal replacement diets, like any other diet plan, should be discussed in detail with a healthcare provider or a qualified dietitian before beginning. They may examine your health situation, decide whether the Cookie Diet is right for you, and offer information on how to utilize it safely.

2. Define your weight loss objectives and set realistic targets for yourself. Remember that many people only try the Cookie Diet for a short period of time because they think it would help them lose weight quickly.

3. Prepare for Success Make sure you have enough of the diet-friendly cookies on hand. Having these cookies on hand is crucial, as they form a key part of the overall strategy.

4. Make a food plan, including what you'll eat for the other meals each day and which ones you'll replace with cookies. A well-balanced meal is permitted on several iterations of the Cookie Diet.

5. Stay hydrated by storing plenty of water and other low-calorie drinks. In addition to improving your health, keeping yourself hydrated might make it easier to resist snacking.

6. Get rid of all the high-calorie, unhealthy snacks and items that could tempt you to break your diet that you found in your kitchen.

Doing so will aid in your ability to stay on track.

7. Setting a routine for when you'll eat your meal replacement cookies and other permitted snacks and drinks is an important step toward sticking to your diet. Adherence can be improved with consistent treatment.

8. One ordinary meal per day (usually dinner) can be included in the Cookie Diet, but if you do, make it a balanced, healthy, and portion-controlled meal. Pick your meals carefully.

9. To maintain tabs on your weight loss efforts, keep a food journal or use a monitoring app to record your daily intake. You can use this to keep on track and make any adjustments.

10. Communicate with loved ones about your diet and ask for their encouragement. Having a group of cheerleaders behind you can help you stay on track.

11. While calorie restriction and meal replacement are at the heart of the Cookie Diet, it's also crucial to make time for regular physical activity. Consistent physical activity can improve outcomes and health in general.

12. Maintain Regular visits with Your Healthcare Provider If your diet plan calls for regular check-ins with a healthcare provider, it is important to keep these visits.

The Cookie Diet, like other meal replacement plans, may not be sustainable in the long run for weight loss. It's typically utilized as a short-term method for quick weight loss. If you want to keep the weight off and improve your health in the long run, you need to switch to a more sustainable and balanced eating plan after you reach your target weight.

Menus for Those on the Cookie Diet

The Cookie Diet, commonly known as "Dr. Siegal's Cookie Diet," is a popular weight-loss plan in which participants replace regular meals with cookie-based meal replacements.

• Use a meal replacement cookie in the morning instead of a real breakfast. These cookies are low in calories while yet packing a healthy punch of protein and fiber to keep hunger at bay.

- At around midday, you may be given another meal replacement cookie or a small, low-calorie snack like raw veggies, fruit, or yogurt, depending on the particular Cookie Diet program you're following.

- For lunch: try having another meal replacement cookie instead of your usual lunch. In order to aid in calorie restriction, these cookies are often sold in predetermined serving sizes.

A meal replacement cookie or other small, low-calorie snack may be appropriate for the afternoon.

Meal: The Cookie Diet allows for a healthy and well-balanced meal in many of its iterations. Grilled chicken, fish, or tofu, as well as a large serving of non-starchy veggies, and a small serving of brown rice or sweet potatoes constitute an ideal nutritious dinner. The goal of this meal is to promote dietary variety and supplement any deficiencies.

Evening Snack: Some variants of the Cookie Diet may include a last meal replacement cookie or a tiny, low-calorie snack as an evening pleasure.

Drinking plenty of water and other low-calorie beverages throughout the day might help you feel fuller for longer and curb cravings.

It's vital to remember that the precise cookie meal plan can change according on the Cookie Diet brand or version you choose, as well as any adaptations made by medical specialists or nutritionists. In addition, the macronutrient and calorie composition of meal replacement cookies can vary widely from product to product, so it's vital to stick to the recommendations made by your particular diet plan.

You should talk to your doctor or a certified dietitian before beginning the Cookie Diet or any meal replacement plan to be sure it will work for your health goals and to learn how to implement it safely and efficiently. For long-term health and weight maintenance, it's best to see the Cookie Diet as a temporary weight-loss method and move on to a more sustainable eating plan.

CHAPTER THREE
Keeping the Weight Off

Maintaining a healthy weight might be as difficult as losing the weight itself. If you've just lost weight and want to keep it off, here are some things to keep in mind.

1. Create Long-Lasting Changes: Make the Change to a Long-Term, Balanced Eating Plan. A wide range of entire foods, including fruits, vegetables, lean meats, whole grains, and healthy fats, are recommended. Avoid starvation or other restrictive diets.

2. Mind your serving sizes to control your weight. When ingested in large quantities, even nutritious meals can cause weight gain. To ensure that your servings are uniform in size, implement instruments like measuring cups or a food scale.

3. Exercise on a Regular Basis: Make working out a regular part of your schedule. Aim for a combination of cardiovascular exercise, strength training, and flexibility exercises. This aids in both weight maintenance and general well-being.

4. Achievable, practical, and long-term targets for weight maintenance should be established.

Keep in mind that it's normal for your weight to go up and down, and that you don't have to be perfect.

5. Keep a food and exercise journal to keep tabs on your progress. Regularly weighing oneself or keeping a meal diary will help you stay accountable and make adjustments when necessary.

6. Always have a strong network of loved ones and friends to fall back on. Tell them about your plans and your progress, and ask for their support when you need it.

7. Hydrate yourself often throughout the day. It's easy to confuse thirst for hunger, which can lead to mindless munching.

8. Focus on what and when you eat in order to practice mindful eating. Eating mindfully can help you tune into your body for signs of hunger and avoid overeating due to stress.

9. Preparation is the key, so plot out your meals and snacks ahead of time. This can help you control your cravings and choose a better option when faced with a similar situation.

10. Indulge in Moderation: Enjoy your favorite delicacies and indulgences in moderation. Cutting out certain types of food from your diet entirely may cause you to binge on others.

11. If you want to stop binge eating, you need to recognize the stresses and emotions that set off your eating disorder. Learn to use positive coping mechanisms to handle your feelings and stress.

12. Check in with a registered dietician or healthcare expert on a regular basis to discuss your progress and receive individualized advice and motivation.

13. Keep Learning: Keep reading up on what you can about healthy food and nutrition. Understanding the nutritional content of meals might help you make more well-rounded decisions.

14. Reduce your stress levels; they can cause you to overeat and gain weight due to emotional eating. Practice stress-reduction methods like meditation, yoga, deep breathing, or enjoyable activities.

15. Sleep Well: Aim for ample and restful sleep. Hormones that control hunger and fullness might be thrown off by a lack of sleep.

16. Acknowledge and celebrate your progress and successes as you work to maintain your weight. Make non-food rewards a priority.

Keep in mind that your efforts to keep the weight off are a lifelong commitment, and that you can expect to experience both highs and lows along the way. Be patient with yourself and be committed to your health and well-being. Maintaining your weight loss can be difficult, so it's important to get help from a healthcare professional or registered dietitian if you're having trouble.

Workouts and Healthiness

Physical activity and fitness are cornerstones of a healthy way of life. The benefits to your body, mind, and spirit from staying physically active and fit are numerous. As a whole, exercise and fitness consist of the following:

Exercise:

• Cardiovascular (aerobic) exercises like running, swimming, and cycling; strength training or resistance exercises using weights or resistance bands; flexibility and mobility exercises like yoga and stretching; and balance exercises are just a few examples of the many types of exercise out there.

2. Gains from Physical Activity:

Physical Health: Exercising regularly can aid in weight control, boost cardiovascular health, lower the risk of chronic diseases (such as heart disease and type 2 diabetes), and increase fitness levels.

• **Mood and Mental Health:** Exercise has been shown to alleviate stress, anxiety, and depression.

Weight-bearing exercises are beneficial to bone and muscle health because they help preserve and even improve bone density and muscle mass.

• **Metabolism:** Exercising frequently can help increase metabolism, which in turn can facilitate weight control.

• **Better Sleep:** Physical activity has been shown to enhance sleep and reduce the severity of sleep disorders.

• The Immune System: Frequent physical activity has been shown to improve the body's defenses against illness.

3. The American Heart Association suggests doing at least 75 minutes of vigorous aerobic activity per week and 150 minutes of moderate aerobic activity, plus doing muscle-strengthening activities at least twice per week. But everyone has different requirements.

Fitness:

1. Components of Physical Fitness There are many different aspects of physical fitness.

The capacity of the heart and lungs to supply oxygen to active muscles is known as cardiovascular endurance.

- **Muscular Strength:** The greatest force that a muscle or muscle group is capable of producing.

Muscular endurance refers to a person's capacity to engage in prolonged muscular contractions.

Range of motion at a joint or set of joints is what we mean when we talk about flexibility.

The ratio of fat to lean mass is known as "body composition."

2. Cardiorespiratory fitness tests (e.g., VO2 max tests), strength assessments, flexibility tests, and body composition measurements are all valid ways to gauge an individual's fitness level.

3. It is common practice to set fitness goals with the intent of enhancing some facet of one's physical well-being. The focus may be on increasing muscular strength, stamina, range of motion, or overall body composition. These objectives serve to inspire and guide physical activity plans.

4. Consistency is the cornerstone of a successful fitness maintenance program. A sustainable fitness routine requires regular exercise, a healthy diet, and plenty of sleep.

5. Fitness should be tailored to each person because everyone has different requirements and objectives. It's important to find an exercise routine that works for you and that you enjoy doing by taking into account your current fitness level, age, health, and personal interests.

If you have any preexisting health conditions or have very specific fitness goals, you should talk to a doctor or fitness expert before beginning any new exercise program. In consultation with them, you can develop a program that is tailored to your specific needs and goals and is both safe and effective.

Conclusion

Physical, mental, and emotional health are all interconnected, making up the full picture of a healthy lifestyle. A healthy diet, regular exercise, and controlling one's weight are all essential. In order to make healthy food choices, one must have a firm grasp on the fundamentals of nutrition, portion control, and eating consciously. Improved cardiovascular health, strength, flexibility, and mental health are just some of the many benefits that come from regular exercise and a focus on physical fitness. In addition, a combination of healthy eating, regular physical activity, and a commitment to long-term change is necessary for effective weight management.

• It's important to approach weight loss and maintenance with a focus on long-term, sustainable habits rather than quick fixes or extreme measures. The keys to achieving and maintaining a healthy lifestyle are creating a supportive environment, seeking advice from healthcare professionals or registered dietitians, remaining motivated, and being patient. You can improve your health, happiness, and quality of life by following these guidelines and making them part of your daily routine.

THE END